Fleur Anderson is a former political journalist and parliamentary sketch writer with the *Australian Financial Review*, ABC's *Insiders* panellist, a past vice-president of the Federal Parliamentary Press Gallery and a founding member of Canberra's Women in Media.

After twenty years in journalism, Fleur Anderson decided to follow Dr Seuss's career advice to go where 'it's opener out there, in the wide open air' to explore the new world of artificial intelligence and digital communication where it's cool to take your dog to the office.

Writers in the *On Series*

Fleur Anderson

On Sleep

hachette
AUSTRALIA

Every attempt has been made to locate the copyright holders for material quoted in this book. Any person or organisation that may have been overlooked or misattributed may contact the publisher.

Published in Australia and New Zealand in 2020
by Hachette Australia
(an imprint of Hachette Australia Pty Limited)
Level 17, 207 Kent Street, Sydney NSW 2000
www.hachette.com.au

First published in 2018 by Melbourne University Publishing

10 9 8 7 6 5 4 3 2 1

 A catalogue record for this book is available from the National Library of Australia

ISBN: 978 0 7336 4402 3 (paperback)

Original cover concept by Nada Backovic Design
Text design by Alice Graphics
Author photograph by Andrew Meares
Typeset by Typeskill
Printed and bound in Australia by McPherson's Printing Group

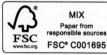 The paper this book is printed on is certified against the Forest Stewardship Council® Standards. McPherson's Printing Group holds FSC® chain of custody certification SA-COC-0053⁷. FSC® promotes environmentally responsible, socially beneficial and economically viable management of the world's forests.

A bedtime story

Once upon a time, a long time ago and in a land far away, there lived a man blessed with such intellect and wit that all those around him knew he was destined for greatness. He, however, had more modest goals: to marry well, to become prime minister and, if he was lucky, to own a racehorse.

Unfortunately, as in all good bedtime stories, there were obstacles. As a young boy, he lost his beloved father and it cast him into such deep despair that his personality changed forever. His reserved nature was mistaken for aloofness. His self-doubt for hesitancy. Where others would quickly overcome slights, he would dwell and stew.

Nevertheless he excelled at university, soaking up knowledge with his cleverness, and in time he succeeded in marrying a well-connected, rich woman. He also bought a horse. Hoorah! With the encouragement of his wife, he entered politics, where he dazzled people with electrifying speeches, clever turns of phrase, his charm and lovely manners. He made his name in foreign affairs, travelling the world as one of his nation's top representatives and urged world cooperation on the day's big issues (while doing his best to advance the interests of his own country). It wasn't long until he had defeated his rivals to become prime minister.

But, of course (remember, this is a bedtime story), he was tormented secretly by the most terrible curse. For every brilliant speech that inspired the crowds, there was an endless night of sleeplessness. Every sparkling public appearance was followed by a debilitating slump of exhaustion. For years in the dark silence of his bedroom, he'd battled the enemies of Nod and, on most nights, had come away the loser. Not even the peace he gained by moving his beloved wife and children into a separate, nearby house/ castle was enough to calm his unruly mind.

Besieged by the constant backstabbing of his Cabinet colleagues and by tawdry rumours about his private life, soon our hero was taking heavy-duty prescription drugs to make it through the night and each following day.

After a minor skirmish in the parliament, our hero quit and took his stunned Cabinet colleagues with him. 'But we could still yet win!' they cried.

'Bugger it,' said our hero. 'I'm too tired for this shit.'[1]

May you rest in peace, Archibald Primrose, fifth Earl of Roseberry, British Prime Minister, March 1894 - June 1895, and patron[2] of sleepless politicians, their families, their staffers, the media that report on them and the public that endure them.

---

1 Not his actual words.
2 Not an actual patron.

Why sleep?

Like a spider perched atop an ant hill, Parliament House crouches on Capital Hill, Canberra. Its web stretches along the avenues and suburbs beneath it. Its silk drifts out, catching some of us irrevocably, while others are only lightly brushed by its touch. It could be any other large organisation—a hospital, a university or a corporate headquarters—in which the daily and nightly lives of the inhabitants are shaped by institutional rhythms. But the political world is different because, to absolutely torture this analogy, it operates under the magnifying glass of the public glare. This scrutiny changes the behaviour of those living under it.

And most of us lie about sleep.

'How are you?'

'Really well, thanks,' we reply. (Oh God, I'm dying inside. I didn't sleep a wink last night. I know it's my own fault and today is going to be a terrible day, the internal monologue goes.) Our sleep is a hidden activity in darkened rooms behind closed doors; we don't parade our peaceful nights like fitness fanatics who boast to the world about their latest running times on social media. (Personal Best last night: 6h 30mins. #8hrssleep goal is in sight!)

Sleep is the most unambitious of pursuits. To sleep is to surrender. As any new parent knows, it's a skill that's both innate and learned. Filled with postpartum hormones and experiencing extreme sleep deprivation, what new parent hasn't had that absolute moment of clarity, realising that the only course of action in the morning is to put their beloved firstborn up for adoption by more capable parents?

For the inmates of Parliament House, the contest between the need for sleep and the demand for public performance is a fascinating spectator sport. Some plod predictably and unremarkably through their many years in the place. Others blaze like a comet through the night—brightly, memorably— and then are gone, as if never there.

For fifteen years, I attended press conferences and interviews in Parliament House and so often wanted to ask the leaders of the time how they slept. 'How do you switch off?' I wanted to ask. Now, after leaving the hothouse of federal political journalism, it's much easier to ask that big question of John Howard, Kevin Rudd, Julie Bishop, Bob Brown and others: 'How do you sleep?'

Why should we care about the sleeping habits of our elected representatives and those who work with them? We need those looking after the running of the country to be at their best, just as we'd expect a pilot or a doctor to be at the peak of their ability, and sleep is integral to our psychological and cognitive wellbeing. In professions where fatigue can have life-or-death consequences, we expect regulations to balance the need for rest against the imperative of delivering profits or results. A 2017 audit by the Australian Medical Association found that more than half of the doctors in Australian public hospitals were working unsafe hours. One doctor reported working an unbroken 76-hour shift, triggering media headlines across the country.[3] Australian airlines are moving to a new 'fatigue risk-management' system that incorporates sleep science into the way airlines manage their day-to-day operations.

In politics, we have codes of conduct, electoral donations, registers for parliamentarians' financial arrangements and, hell, even a 'bonk ban' outlining who can 'sleep' with whom. But workplace guidelines to ensure adequate sleep? Don't be soft. Politics is for the hard men and women of this world. It is where clever plans are hatched in late-night rendezvous in Chinese restaurants, where

---

3 Roje Adaimy, 'Half of hospital doctors work "unsafe hours", audit reveals', AAP, 15 July 2017.

careers are built and destroyed by working the phones when the meek choose to sleep.

Parliament is the most visible and exaggerated example of how our society is changing. It illustrates the blurring of our daytime work hours into night, the impact of technology on the 24/7 media cycle, and the slow twisting and shaping of our biological sleep patterns to fit our modern lives. In a democracy, parliament is our society's last line of defence, safeguarding our wellbeing, our pursuit of happiness. In some far-off future, it may be our democracy that decides what it means to be human.

Regardless of their protestations at election time, politicians never have been, nor will they ever be, 'normal' people. Personal and ideological ambition drives them harder than the rest of us. And thank goodness for that. Can you imagine a country governed by people who quit the school parents' association after a term because of the internecine warfare between the tuckshop volunteers and the fete committee?

Yet we need our elected representatives to remain connected to our everyday rhythms—of waking in the pale dawn to gently prod our children awake, the morning commute, the early evening conflict of a trip to the gym versus a wine or two, a late-night work email check, or the start of the late shift on a second job. Until technology intervenes to 'cure' our need for sleep, this is our life in the twenty-first century.

In the beginning

One Saturday night during the 2016 federal election, sleep and I hit a rocky patch. As a Canberra-based journalist for *The Australian Financial Review*, I'd started appearing the previous year on the ABC's Sunday-morning political television show, *Insiders*. It's filmed in Melbourne, and due to the early start, all non-Victorian panellists fly there on Saturday evening.

From previous experience, I had my routine down pat. My kit consisted of the weekend's newspapers, a week of political media clippings, a set of freshly pressed, television-appropriate clothes, a notebook, a bottle of low-dose kava tablets from the health-food store to keep hyperactive thoughts at bay, a toothbrush and toothpaste. Checking into the comfortable serviced apartments across the road from the ABC's Southbank studios, I found the room identical to those of previous visits. I knew where the kettle and teabags were kept and how to use the microwave and TV. I'd stayed there only a fortnight earlier for a previous show. Easy.

I settled in for an early night. A single-serve bottle of low-alcohol wine and a frozen dinner from the local supermarket around the corner, while I made some quick hand-written notes on recent events and my observations of the political week. Phone alarm set for 6.30 a.m. So sensible. No pre-appearance nerves for me!

Like all good horror stories, it begins innocently enough. As I am drifting off in the plush sheets with better pillows than the lumpy old things at home, the air-conditioning unit suddenly rumbles to life. Stumbling around in the dark to find the air-conditioning control, I manage to turn it off. Outside there are the usual late-night sounds of pub drinkers noisily returning home, cars passing and the occasional siren. Another peaceful night in the city.

The air-conditioning unit starts again. *Clunk, thunk, bang.* And again. And again, the discordant racket steadily evolving into words, into lyrics of midnight wakefulness. '*Clunk-thunk-bang*-nev-er-sleep-nev-er-sleep.' Like Edgar Allan Poe's Raven chanting 'nevermore', my air-conditioning unit has attained sentience.

And—apologies to Poe—it has to be *this* midnight dreary, while I am weak and weary.

Realising finally that a neighbouring room's unit is making the noise, I think, Hmmm, annoying, and return to bed.

But the damage is done. What was that thing Barnaby Joyce said about trade tariffs? Do I need to brush up on the latest on the government's industrial relations policies? What on earth is going on with Victorian Labor's factional battles, and what can I say about them that hasn't been said before? To put my mind at rest, I turn on the computer to work for a few minutes in bed. (Ah yes, breaking the first rules of good sleep hygiene, you think to yourself. You know what's coming next, just like when an actor in a slasher movie says, 'I'm just going to see what that screaming noise is in the attic.')

Once more on the cusp of sleep, a leg twitches violently. Wide awake again and immediately wondering what I can say with any conviction about Australia's energy security and the likelihood of an effective emissions-trading scheme, I check the clock. Two-fifteen a.m. Quarter past two. Four hours and fifteen minutes until the alarm goes off. It is a quarter past panic o'clock. Politics is no longer keeping me awake. Worrying about not sleeping is keeping me awake.

What follows is embarrassing. Three cycles of 'Salute to the Sun' yoga while the sun is still hours away. Manically performed meditation exercises while listening to a free downloaded phone app called 'Self-Hypnosis for Weight Loss and Relaxation'. Tensing and relaxing muscles while imagining a stroll through a terraced orange orchard, 'with each level lower taking you to a new level of relaxation'. Or not.

Sleep seems almost within reach as I listen to a white noise app combining the sounds of rain and thunder—until I jolt with a start. Have I plugged in the phone charger? What if the phone runs out of battery and the alarm doesn't come on? What if I don't wake up? If I die, will the *Insiders* crew break into my hotel room to check? Will my lifeless body be discovered with my mouth open and dried drool on my cheek? Oh God. I'm wearing my worst nightie.

Shortly before dawn I give up. I shower and pack my bags: newspapers, notebooks, my useless bottle of relaxation-inducing herbal tablets. I make the bed and lie on top of it to wait out those last hours in that hated prison cell of a room … and wake up at 7 a.m. with the phone alarm blaring. An hour and a half's sleep! I feel like punching the air in jubilation.

The make-up artists repair my ravaged face and hair. The show begins, and my profound midnight thoughts on the state of the world flow effortlessly from my mouth. With the slow-motion focus of the slightly drunk, I watch host Barrie Cassidy interview Foreign Minister Julie Bishop live from Perth, becoming momentarily fixated by the way she pronounces 'Daesh' and 'to'. It doesn't even occur to me to wonder how someone like Bishop could look as alert and collected at 6 a.m. in Perth as she does at 2 p.m. at Question Time in Canberra. Instead I am preoccupied and exhilarated by the delusional idea that I—for one—no longer need sleep.

Sleep discovery

There's no shortage of expert advice on getting a good night's sleep. A growing mountain of evidence from uncomfortable experiments on dogs, mice and jellyfish will soon solve the mystery of why we must be unconscious and vulnerable for a third of our lives. Or so we are told.

Later I discover my midnight torture in that apartment was probably due to the so-called 'First Night Effect': the phenomenon where sleeping in an unfamiliar place prompts one hemisphere of the brain to go on sentry duty. It's a remnant of our prehistoric evolution. During the first night in a new place, a small part of the left hemisphere remains active and sensitive to sounds even during the deepest phases of sleep. It's good to know we'll still hear a sabre-toothed tiger, even in a secure inner-city serviced apartment.

But that's not much comfort at 3 a.m. when you can't switch off. It's just too bloody late for all the 'fail-safe' sleep remedies: take a magnesium pill, quit coffee, quit alcohol, 'live your best life'. At 3 a.m., the only resources to hand are internet cat videos and a reservoir of regret and self-loathing for bingeing on wine and pizza and making our spouses' lives a misery with our sleep-deprived, toxic-lifestyle snoring.

Why can't we learn from those hours of uninterrupted introspection? Where are the stories about the times sleeplessness led to life-changing decisions? Why don't we appreciate those dark hours without the constant chatter of waking life, when we are free to consider our flaws and mistakes? When we have that moment where creativity strikes and we can't wait for the sun to rise so we can put our crazy/brave plans into action? When we decide in the silence of our bedrooms that 'from now on, I'm going to do things differently'? When a night of sleeplessness changes history?

When I'm in the middle of the Midnight Frets, I want to know that there are other people—the successful, the wealthy, the healthy and the rest of us—awake as well. And that on this night, for whatever reason, we're not going to sleep but tomorrow we'll still be okay. Who are these fellow insomniacs? You can't find the answers in Hansard or in the media reports of the day. But it is possible to ask, and it's surprising how often people will tell you the truth.

The politics of sleep

'How do you sleep at night?' It's a pejorative question—often shouted through megaphones at rallies about refugee policy, climate change or war. No wonder public figures are reluctant to engage. For public figures, there's a professional risk in talking about sleep. Admit having too much of it and people will think a politician is lying or deluded. Admit to too little sleep and voters will still think the same, with an added worry about the politicians being medically unsafe to operate the heavy machinery of government.

On the night Australia celebrated the end of the long journey to legalising marriage equality, the ABC's *7.30* presenter Leigh Sales asked Malcolm Turnbull how he'd been sleeping. With the ongoing drama of the dual citizenship scandal just the latest head-ache of the Turnbull prime ministership, it was reasonable to assume there'd been some sleepless nights:

LEIGH SALES: Prime Minister, what runs through your head in the middle of the night when you wake up and you can't sleep?

MALCOLM TURNBULL: You know what? I sleep right through the night. Do you sleep well?

LEIGH SALES: No, I wake up often in the night, which is why I assume everybody does. I'm sure you don't sleep through every night.

MALCOLM TURNBULL: You would be amazed. The key to being a happy and effective prime minister is to get a good night's sleep and plenty of exercise.

Hang on a second. What? Like many people watching, I didn't believe for a minute the Prime Minister, or in fact any prime minister, could sleep through the night. His refusal to admit to sleepless nights could only be for fear of displaying a weakness to be exploited by critics both inside and outside his government. 'I sleep through the night' had the same ring of inauthenticity as Julia Gillard's claim during her prime ministership that she, progressive and feminist, didn't support same-sex marriage. It seemed an answer driven by politics, rather than truth.

But discussing the Turnbull interview the next day, a friend—a relatively high-profile executive—was surprised that anyone would even doubt the PM's claim that he sleeps well at night. 'Oh, I believed him,' she said. 'I sleep eight hours every night, no matter what. Don't you?' My friend certainly always looks well rested—the whites of her eyes still possessing that slightly glowing, bluish tinge of childhood, compared with the dark circles and spidery red lines snaking through the whites of non-sleepers.

Could it be true? Could there be two races of superhuman: one whose secret strength is the ability to get their full complement of eight hours every night, 'no matter what';

and the other who can get by on only an hour or two whenever they have to?

Actually I'm half right, according to sleep expert Dr Carmel Harrington. There *are* two secret groups of superhumans—but not quite like I'd imagined.

Any fan of the 1980s horror flick *The Fly* will not be surprised that all the trouble starts when scientists tinker with the genetics of flies—wild fruit flies, or *Drosophila melanogaster*, to be exact. They find that some flies can live on only a little sleep with no impairment of their abilities, while others need more sleep than average to operate at full capacity. The researchers discovered that the sleep requirements of flies are a family trait, and before you know it, scientists are looking for evidence of short-sleeping fruit fly genes in human family trees. Or something like that.

It turns out that about 3 per cent of the human population need on average two hours' less sleep a night than the rest of us. Let's call them the super-awake. And another 3 per cent of the population are the super-sleepers, who need an extra two hours' sleep to function normally. And the average person? We need about seven to nine hours a night to be at our superhero best.

We all know at least one of these super-awake people, particularly in politics and business. They tend to be very active, often with an extra job or extracurricular activities.

And they tend to be slim without trying hard. How deeply irritating.

The rest of us can only pretend to be so genetically blessed. But there are huge pitfalls in kidding ourselves that we don't need much sleep. Dr Harrington is an expert speaker who frequently addresses blue-chip chief executives, law firms, accounting groups and health providers, for which risk management is core business. Here's the bit she tells them that scares the pants off in-house legal teams.

A recent experiment compared the effects of sleep deprivation in two groups: one group was permitted to sleep only six hours a night for two weeks, and another group was kept awake for three nights. The no-sleep-for-three-nights group naturally reported feeling very tired and miserable. The restricted sleep group reported feeling pretty tired for the first couple of days but then not that bad after the two weeks[4]

Here's the thing: both groups showed almost the exact level of impairment in physical, working memory and cognitive performance. What's more, the acute–sleep deprivation group knew they couldn't perform to standard, but the six-hour-a-night group were unaware they were so impaired. In fact, another study of financial decision-making by the chronically and acutely tired showed

---

4 Carmel Harrington, 'Chronic sleep deprivation and its connection with distraction', National Road Safety Partnership Program, www.nrspp.org.au; Hans P.A. Van Dongen, Greg Maislin, Janet M. Mullington and David F. Dinges, 'The cumulative cost of additional wakefulness: Dose-response effects on neurobehavioral functions and sleep physiology from chronic sleep restriction and total sleep deprivation', *Sleep*, 15 March 2006, vol. 26, no. 2, pp. 117–26.

that people who'd had their sleep restricted by only a couple of hours a night were more likely to engage in risky behaviour, compared with people who stayed up all night and knew they were tired.[5]

Not long ago, Dr Harrington spoke to an audience of surgeons and asked them to take part in an anonymous electronic audience survey. 'Do any of you think you've made a serious error due to lack of sleep?' she asked. 'Yes' was the response from 90 per cent of the audience. Now, let's think about that: nine out of ten surgeons (albeit in a single small room) believed they'd made a serious mistake in their professional life due to tiredness. Let's not react with condemnation because— given the opportunity of anonymity—they at

5 Harrington, 'Chronic sleep deprivation'.

least were aware of their own fallibility. I'm not sure I could say the same.

Now let's consider the impact of sleep deprivation on our ability to distinguish right from wrong. A study of people in a raffle ticket competition found participants were more likely to cheat if they'd had as little as twenty-two minutes' less sleep than normal. Another study found we're less likely to search the internet for ethics-related queries the day we shift our clocks forward to daylight-saving time. Other studies found tired people are less likely to notice unethical behaviour in others, or even to recognise in the first place whether there is a moral or ethical question at stake.[6]

6 Gauri Sarda-Joshi, 'How does sleep loss affect your view of right and wrong?', *Sleep Junkies*, 6 April 2018, <https://sleepjunkies.com/science/sleep-morality-ethical-behavior>.

When I speak to Dr Harrington, the Australian cricket team is in deep disgrace for ball tampering. For the time being, it seems the professional career of the captain, Steve Smith, is in tatters for his decision to cheat in that match against South Africa. A year earlier, Smith had asked the Dalai Lama for the secret of a good night's sleep.[7] 'I asked him a question about sleep and how he could help me—he gave me his blessings, we rubbed our noses together,' Smith said. 'Hopefully it will help me with my sleep over the next five days.' It obviously didn't work for long because in December 2017, he had to take a sleeping pill the night before Australia

---

7 Andrew Wu, 'Australia captain Steve Smith to sleep easier after personal meeting with Dalai Lama', *The Sydney Morning Herald*, 24 March 2017.

won the second Ashes test in Adelaide. Did Smith still struggle with sleep during that ill-fated tour of South Africa? 'This is the guy who is entering the zone. This is the guy who can't sleep,' said veteran sports writer Robert 'Crash' Craddock in the aftermath of the cricket scandal. If he was struggling, Smith is obviously not the only one making question-able decisions with a tired brain.

In the 1960s, a major study on the early indicators of cancer also found that adults were getting an average of 8.5 hours' sleep. Today, the average sleep for a working adult is 6.8 hours. 'As biological beings, we haven't changed our needs that much,' Dr Harrington says. If all this research is to be believed, we should all be frightened out of our wits. We're short-changing ourselves, but on the upside, we have on average an extra 1.7 hours a day to binge-watch Netflix, and to check Facebook, Twitter and Instagram updates. I once spent an entire insomniac night reading a five-year-old blog thread on the history of terrine-making. Who says Western civilisation is in decline?

We've become a society of the chronically overtired. So tired, we don't realise we're mentally impaired. So tired that we don't recognise risky decisions. So tired that we don't notice unethical behaviour in others or ourselves. So exhausted that we don't even realise there's a moral question in front of us.

Into the Forgettory

It was difficult to discern over the phone, but I'm guessing that momentary pause—after I'd asked Kevin Rudd, Australia's twenty-sixth prime minister, whether it was true he slept less than three hours a night—was actually a frustrated sigh and an invisible eye roll. 'It always stuns me: the capacity for the media to continue to misreport given my multiple corrections of that particular story,' he said. En route to Perth Airport in the pre-dawn hours to catch a flight to Munich, Rudd's voice revealed no signs of early-morning croakiness or even the 4.15 a.m.

crankiness suffered by us mere mortals before an early international flight.

We'd tried to make contact the afternoon before he left Melbourne, after a lightning visit back to Australia to commemorate the tenth anniversary of 'the Apology' to the Stolen Generations. But somehow we'd missed each other, what with international mobile phone numbers, unfamiliar country number prefixes and strange phone diversions to automated international answering services. I'd planned to ask him about his much-reported short sleeping hours. Instead I was the one who'd stayed awake that night, berating myself for being unable to use international phone numbers and for embarrassing my contacts who had helped facilitate the interview, sure that my children and their children's children would be forever cursed for being related to 'that woman who couldn't work a phone properly'.

'That particular story', as he called it when we did finally speak, was from an interview with his wife, Thérèse Rein, who'd said her husband could operate on three hours' sleep and had always been able to do so since she'd met him at university.[8] He characterised it as 'a throw-away line' delivered 'in a light-hearted way'. But there's no getting past the stories that have emerged from friends and foes, politicians and public servants, of a prime minister who appeared to operate around the clock.

8 Annabel Crabb, '3 hours' sleep is all the PM needs', *The Sydney Morning Herald*, 18 July 2009.

'So what's the truth?' he asks, a classic Rudd rhetorical question. 'The truth is each night I will try to get anywhere between six and eight hours' sleep. And for me, I function okay on six hours, and I function well on seven, and eight is damned comfortable.'

I mention that some people have no trouble dropping off when it's time to sleep, while others, like me, lie there forever thinking about how to sleep. 'Not the product of a troubled soul, I hope,' he says. Rudd, like many of those with whom I've had similar conversations, has his doubts about those urban myths of leaders and geniuses who can operate on scant sleep.

Literally since Thomas Edison invented the light bulb, we've been deceiving ourselves about our sleep. Sleeping eight to ten hours a day? It's the habit of a caveman, Edison proclaimed. Those who went to bed with the chickens, rising at dawn with the roosters, were dullards compared with those illuminated by the white-hot filaments of the electric age. It's no coincidence, then, that Edison's friends helpfully snapped photographs on their box Brownies of Edison's daytime napping in parks, on laboratory benches and in front of US presidents. No one likes a blowhard.

In his post-parliament life, Rudd's happy to admit sometimes there's a deficit between the hours of sleep needed to function at full capacity and the hours you actually get. As prime minister or foreign minister, sleep is a problem of logistics as 'you are ripping yourself from one side of the continent to the other and in and out of time zones'.

In the win-at-all-costs world of politics, reports of scant sleep by leaders are often used for political ends by their opponents. Barack Obama was often reported to sleep anywhere between three and six hours a night. Margaret Thatcher got four hours a night. Donald Trump is also a reported four-to-five-hour sleeper, and his midnight tweet in 2017 about 'negative press covfefe' triggered a wave of internet memes and speculation that the leader of the free world may be suffering from chronic sleep deprivation. Rudd himself was reported to have slept only one hour (in an armchair) during the marathon forty-hour 2009 Copenhagen Accord on climate change—'one of the greatest moral, economic and environmental challenges of our age'—and was rather testy as a result.[9]

Humans tend to be beasts who favour biphasic sleep patterns: a long sleep of five to seven hours at night, followed by a fifteen–ninety-minute nap in the afternoon. By economic necessity, we've evolved to be monophasic—sleeping a long stretch at night, followed by a quick trip to the chocolate bar–vending machine at 3 p.m. in lieu of an afternoon nap. The siesta survives in some countries—including Greece, Italy, Spain, the Philippines, Costa Rica and Mexico (all of them with hot climates)—but sadly not in Australia. Perhaps our weekday afternoons would be a more relaxed affair had Australia been colonised by the Spanish.

---

9 David Marr, 'We need to talk about Kevin … Rudd, that is', *The Sydney Morning Herald*, 7 June 2010.

By political necessity, leaders often seem to revert to ancient polyphasic sleep patterns, also championed by Silicon Valley types who trade Bulletproof coffee formulas to really get the heart going. By discarding a large block of sleep, the normal transitional phases of sleep can be abandoned, saving time for just the slow-wave REM sleep in multiple twenty-minute bursts throughout a 24-hour period. So restful! Don't we feel great!

More difficult for the rest of us to reconcile is how any sleep can come in that unimaginable, incandescent glare of public life where your actions, your history, your very psyche are dissected publicly by friend and foe. And where it's your own colleagues who can cut the deepest. 'The bottom line is it's an intense era of public life,' Rudd says of his experience of prime ministership. 'As soon as you're out in the public domain and no longer a private person, there is an entirely different part of your brain activated, where everything you think, say and do is public property. That's a whole new reality for people.'

Reading an unexciting book, meditating or giving up coffee can only go so far in getting you off to sleep when you are coping with the feelings of injustice and—let's be honest—rage when you've been publicly criticised without an avenue for rebuttal. How often do we relive moments of heartfelt praise from others? Once? Twice? Or not at all because our cruel biology compels us to rehash the negative?

There's a lovely French phrase to describe the regret of not saying the right thing at the right time: *l'esprit de l'escalier*—'staircase wit', thinking of the reply too late, when we are already halfway down or up the staircase. And, of course, our memories are at their photographic best in the midnight hours as we remember *that thing* we should have said to *that person* when they said it *that time*. Even author J.K. Rowling has fallen prey to the mind's cruel trick of keeping us awake, and then replaying our past humiliations in technicolour glory. She tweeted:

> You develop excellent recall when you wake at 4am to relive that stupid thing you said on the evening of June 8th 1994, while Ace of Base were playing on the radio in the kitchen with the blue worktops and the crooked Venetian blind. Or so I'd imagine.[10]

---

10 J.K. Rowling, Twitter, 2 March 2018.

So how do we ease our subconscious mind, which inconveniently revives our old regrets, past grievances and midnight staircase wit? 'I think there is a discipline about going to sleep and I don't know if it works more generally for people, but for me, it's got two parts to it,' Rudd says. The first is to distinguish the things you can and cannot control, to reconcile them and hopefully stop your mind returning automatically to those things that are, as Rudd says, 'outside your purchase'.

'The second thing is forgiveness.' It's here we take a deep dive into spirituality, into a world of prayer, of self-reflection, of the recognition of being part of something bigger than yourself, of God, of Buddha, of Hinduism, of the meditative qualities of the prayer of St Francis of Assisi. Not being a particularly spiritual person, I don't have much to contribute to this—and I suspect it shows.

'What I'm saying is nothing to do with formal religion; it's to do with spirituality, and it doesn't have a particular ritualistic form—namely to enter into a particular place, to enter a particular space—although churches, as inevitably beautiful and quiet places … can restore salve to the soul,' Rudd explains.

Which brings us to 'the Forgettory' as handed down as canon in the Rudd–Rein family tradition. The Forgettory, Rudd explains, is a place where you put the hurts and slights from people you have forgiven for delivering them to you. 'The best mental image you can have is those ancient computer software programs where they would literally pick out a piece of the text and then transport it using a sucking device from your computer screen and then [dump it] into the rubbish bin,' he says. 'That's putting it into the Forgettory. It's that mental image that I think is important.'

The alternative, he says, is a lifetime accumulation of psychological scar tissue from people who have said terrible things or done terrible things to you. 'I mean, in my case, I would've had to have carried around a walking cross-referenced *Encyclopædia Britannica* to keep track of it all,' he says. So, in Rudd's words, the process is first to engage with the person who done you wrong, second to set the record straight, third to forgive, and then fourth to stick it in the Forgettory. If you don't, then all you are left with is 'a bucket of simmering hatreds' that stop you getting to sleep, he says.

Were there any specific times when sleep deprivation led to poor outcomes or bad decisions during his time in politics? He says, with that quiet, measured Ruddian delivery, 'I think where I've seen it most actively is [in] the inherent stupidities of the Australian parliamentary democracy, where this false macho culture of sitting late into the night in the parliament or into the early morning to pass such critical legislation [means] that we had to threaten each other with a Mexican standoff, revolvers pointed to each other's heads, in a rolling game of Russian Roulette, where the real leverage is sleep. And you just want to get out of there.' Clearly not everything makes it into the Forgettory.

Sleeping for Australia

Julie Bishop is an excellent sleeper. That is, she excels at sleeping when she does it—which is not particularly often. For almost five years as Australia's foreign minister and almost the same period before that as shadow foreign minister, Bishop attributes her ability to be sharp on a handful of hours' sleep to good genes and strict discipline.

Like athletes and other overachievers from big families, who hone their competitive edge as children by fighting for food, toys and attention, perhaps the fight for family commodities—including sleep—has shaped her sleep resilience. 'It could have something to do with the fact that as a little girl I shared a room with my two older sisters and they were very good sleepers,' she says.

It's almost a week until Christmas, and instead of winding down for the holiday break, Bishop finishes her year with yet another punishing, time-bending work week. As a Perth-based federal politician dealing with a three-hour time difference with Canberra, Bishop's sleeping hours are shaped as much by geography as by her occupation. At the Hague or the UN, a chat about sleep or lack of it is a diplomatic icebreaker for the world's foreign ministers, as mundane as discussing the weather is for the rest of us. How was the flight? How did you sleep? What route did you take? How about that snowstorm? New hotels, consecutive nights sleeping on planes, delayed flights and lost luggage are all part of a foreign minister's lot. Bishop and her New Zealand counterpart have by far the most arduous and lengthy trips of most foreign ministers—and on commercial flights rather than the government jets favoured by European and North American foreign ministers.

Yet the challenge of performing in public office on very little sleep is a common theme for this elite group. Hillary Clinton, the most well-travelled secretary of state in US history, complained in released emails that when it comes to sleep, she didn't 'get enough of it, always want more of it,' and that she'd like to go to 'one of those Swiss sleep sanitariums if they still exist'. Former French foreign minister Laurent Fabius was caught on camera nodding off, waking, smiling and dozing again for more than a minute during a business meeting in Algiers. And former mayor and current British foreign minister Boris Johnson has boasted that he only needs four hours' sleep, just like Baroness Margaret Thatcher, prompting some to suggest he try to have more sleep, and maybe a better diet as well.

As for Bishop? Her fitness regime and mental toughness are well known. When I suggest maybe those northern hemisphere foreign ministers should quit their bitching about their travel and jet lag, she laughs. Obviously the thought may have crossed her mind. Forget about Fitbits or smart devices measuring the quality and quantity of her sleep, or the sleep medicine voodoo demanding the 'princess and the pea' mattress toppers favoured by professional jetsetting athletes.

The only technology she allows into her sleep routine is her mobile phone, permanently switched on and lying on the bedside table in case something happens somewhere in the rest of the world. Bishop says she's never experienced the 'First Night Effect', perhaps because after almost a decade in the foreign affairs portfolio, every night is a 'first night'. 'Somehow I've managed to train myself to keep one ear open to listen just in case I need to take a call,' she says. It immediately brings to mind one of those old Looney Tunes cartoons of Bugs Bunny or Road Runner sleeping with one eye open, ever vigilant for the latest antics of Wile E. Coyote or Elmer Fudd. The reality is much more grim. 'I can assure you that as foreign minister, if my phone rings at 2 a.m., it's rarely good news,' she says.

Thanks to her commitment to 6 a.m. runs, regardless of where she is in the world, Bishop says she doesn't get jet lag and she doesn't get sick. 'No,' she corrects herself. 'Actually, only once, I think, in the five years I've been doing this job, I only recall one instance where lack of sleep and coming down with the flu combined to … well, I ended up coming down with pneumonia.'

That one instance was the aftermath of the downing of Malaysia Airlines MH17 over Ukraine on 17 July 2014. 'I was in London and it was just nonstop, unrelenting, and I came down with flu, which then became pneumonia and I had to go see a doctor in London,' Bishop says. Where most of us might consider illness and foreign medical systems as candidates for a dinner-party collection of Worst Travel Stories, Bishop's admission sounds almost like a confession.

And it's understandable. We expect our politicians and public figures to be *just like us*; that is, until they admit to being tired, run-down or—the very worst—bored. Perhaps it's a reflection of our nation's tall poppy syndrome, or maybe we simply want those who represent us to represent only the very best of us, not our day-to-day selves who also get tired or sick or cranky. None of us is perfect, but our representatives must be perfection personified: of unwavering good judgement and with a superhuman body and mind. They must also be capable of perfect restorative sleep, except when we demand them to work for us around the clock.

For Bishop, it wasn't just the responsibility of representing Australia in our moment of genuine national outrage and fury about the bombing of a routine commercial flight over an unremarkable field in Ukraine. She was also carrying a personal burden of grief at the murder of her own constituents, the Maslin family, who lost their three children, Mo, Evie and Otis, and their grandfather Nick Norris, as well as the deaths of thirty-nine Australians from almost every state.

Her role prosecuting Australia's demands for justice for the victims of the MH17 bombing remains the defining moment of Bishop's public life to date. It no doubt took a private toll as well—she was in regular contact with many of the victims' families, and with her own department officials on the ground in Ukraine as they battled to secure the crash zone so the murdered Australians' remains could be repatriated. And then there was the looming shadow of Russia, the task of trying to convince Vladimir Putin to use his influence to allow investigators back to the crash site so they could continue trying to identify the victims before the northern winter descended. Finally, a snatch of sleep here or there was no longer enough. It was pneumonia and exhaustion that brought her down.

But in Australia, we were none the wiser: the foreign minister was merely in transit. 'I slept all the way home,' she says. 'I became sick in London, but then I had the flight from London to Dubai—about seven hours—and then Dubai to Perth, which is about ten hours. I slept all the way. By the time I got back to Perth, I was pretty much better.'

In a continent as large as Australia, the demands of sleep and work do not stop for travelling politicians. The day before I speak to Bishop, she has spent the day in her WA seat of Curtin. As deputy Liberal leader, she takes part in the daily leadership teleconference call, which begins at 7 a.m. on the east coast. Which is, of course, 4 a.m. in the west. Her last electorate event finished at 10.15 p.m., just in time to catch the 10.50 p.m. flight from Perth to Melbourne, 'the Midnight Horror' Bishop fondly calls it. Sometime early Wednesday morning, she caught another flight to Canberra, just in time for Prime Minister Malcolm Turnbull's latest ministerial reshuffle. In the official pictures taken that morning at Government House, Bishop looks as sharp as her well-tailored Armani suits. 'I'm still operating,' she says a few hours later. 'I've probably had two hours' sleep. I'm okay.' By this stage, it's mid-afternoon and hot, at a time of year when many workers are fighting drowsily to make it through those last few hours after the office Christmas lunch. Bishop, however, does sound 'okay'; in fact, you'd never know she hadn't slept.

That night after we speak, Bishop boards the plane to Perth, arriving around ten o'clock Perth time (1 a.m. Eastern Standard Time). The following morning she will probably be up at 6 a.m. (Perth time) for her usual hour-long morning run because, as she says, in her time zone–trained brain, 'it's morning! It's time to go for a run!'

Sleep seems an undemanding pet in the life of a foreign minister. During the week, it gets the bare minimum of attention between the demands of work and travel. The weekends are when it demands she make up for lost time. 'Hopefully, tomorrow night, or Friday night, I'll have time to catch up on a bit more sleep,' Bishop says cheerfully.

Sleeping in public

It takes a certain confidence to catnap. That you'll wake from a twenty-minute nap refreshed, sparkly eyed and without telltale creases on the cheek. To sleep in public, however, requires either extreme exhaustion or next-level chutzpah.

Julie Bishop can't do it, but Kevin Rudd and John Howard are skilled catnappers. So is former *Huffington Post* editor Tory Maguire, who, armed with the authority of sleep revolutionary and *HuffPost* founder Arianna Huffington, set up a 'nap room' in the outfit's Australian headquarters. No bigger than a large broom cupboard, it held an unfashionable recliner and had maybe enough room for one person to do a downward dog. Maguire, working long hours as the inaugural Australian editor, made it a daily ritual to retire to the nap room each afternoon, set her phone timer for seventeen minutes and, without fail, achieve a refreshing afternoon snooze. But only a handful of employees used it. 'Don't use it,' one employee's wary spouse warned. 'It's a management trick to test you.'

As habitual catnappers point out, their habit is less time-consuming and less costly to the taxpayer than the smokers clustered outside buildings on 'smoko'. Some Parliament House old hands, working in open-plan offices, positioned their desks so that a quick under-desk nap could be performed without discovery. It sounded like a delightful idea until rumours got around about a flea infestation in the parliamentary carpet caused by rats and mice on their nocturnal scamperings through the building.

Then there are the public sleepers, those parkour practitioners of catnapping. Asleep on floors in airport terminals, on buses and trains, and, heartbreakingly, on busy footpaths that serve as makeshift beds for the growing number of homeless in our major cities. Every now and then, there's the social awkwardness of 'close personal proximity' sleepers, returning jet-lagged on international flights or an early-morning flight home from a buck's weekend.

A few years ago, returning with my husband to Canberra on an early Sunday-morning flight from the Gold Coast, a youngish man in a black suit took his seat across the aisle. Within minutes of take-off, his chin dipped to his chest and a small drip of claggy liquid emerged from his left nostril. Big night, we nodded to ourselves. Quickly, however, that small drip grew. At first like an icicle. Then longer and longer, swaying in and out with each quiet breath, almost but not quite touching his lips. My husband poked me, 'Look at him now'. The man was breathing deeply and regularly, his breath catching the horror from his nose like a south-easterly filling a large, diaphanous spinnaker. It stretched past his chin, drifting perilously close to his silk tie.

Having had a rather late night myself at a wedding the previous day, I gagged and had to stare straight ahead, although the billowing horrible thing remained at the corner of my eye. Was he another wedding guest returning home, still wearing the suit from the night before? We didn't recognise him. Or maybe he'd been at a funeral. Or a property development conference. Maybe he had SARS.

By this stage, the flight attendants had noticed the disaster unfolding in row 24. Their matt-lipstick smiles remained fixed, but as they passed, their eyes widened in fright. A hurried, furtive conversation at the front of the plane. We tried to read their lips. 'There's a sleeping man at the back with a huge snot hanging out of his nose.'

'Which one? Oh God! I see it! What should we do?'

We watched a flight attendant approach with a wad of thick paper napkins. In a carefully timed manoeuvre to avoid the wet curtain blowing in and out, she efficiently arranged the napkins under his chin and on his lap. The attendant smiled a grim, close-lipped not-smile as she continued on her way.

It was an hour-and-a-half flight and the suspense grew. What would happen first: would he wake to discover the napkins and the thing from his nose, or would he sleepily swat this thing flapping over his face? It was the latter. Still asleep, he swatted it, spreading it across his face. Minutes later, the plane bumped onto the runway and the man awoke to the napkins and all the wet ghastliness of the past hour and a half. We all looked politely away, removing our cabin bags and not meeting each other's eyes. 'Have a great weekend,' the attendant chirped.

Our sleeping hours are our most vulnerable time. Mouths open, drool spilling, involuntary farting, eyeballs darting under eyelids in the most disconcerting way. Then there's the snoring. The horn blast of an ocean liner is nothing compared with me. Our sleeping selves are the opposite of what we wish people to see. Stay awake and stay in control.

Switching off

It was 24 February 2017, 8.30 a.m. Sabra Lane, presenter of ABC Radio's flagship current affairs program, *AM*, sat still and silent in a darkened studio in Parliament House. The last live political interview for the week, with Labor's Shadow Attorney-General Mark Dreyfus, was done. But instead of gathering her papers and leaving that dark, sound-proof room for the high-energy banter of the newsroom outside, Lane sat motionless.

That morning, the studio webcams, installed overhead so interstate producers can monitor studio operations, captured the back of the presenter's head as her shoulders slumped and her chin sank to her chest. 'Sabra, are you okay?' a voice from the Sydney control room asked in her headphones. After a moment, she shook her head. No. Not okay. Lane, an accomplished and experienced political presenter, had only minutes before thanked her audience for listening, wished them a good weekend and—after a morning of on-air stumbles and tongue tangles—promised them that 'hopefully I won't be so stumble-y next week'. It was an uncharacteristic admission from the presenter of a normally slick live current affairs program.

'Get out of the studio now. Go straight to your phone because I'm calling you right now,' her producer said. Still struggling to speak, Lane answered the phone. 'You are upset with yourself because you think you had a really bad week, aren't you?' the producer said.

Lane, previously ABC's *7.30* political editor, was a few weeks into the new gig, which requires 4 a.m. starts each day, as well as late-afternoon and early-evening prerecorded interviews. This week, sleep had taken a back seat to the demands of covering the first fractious fortnight of federal parliament for 2017 as well as monitoring developments in Western Australia, complicated by the associated three-hour time zone difference. 'Yes,' she said in tears to her producer. 'I was really bad.'

'Don't you dare,' he interrupted her. An on-air stumble is an occupational hazard for professional broadcasters. Getting upset about the wobbles creates a domino effect, shaking the confidence of even the best of them. Plus there was no time for self-pity. Two-term WA Liberal Premier Colin Barnett was on the ropes, and the relationship between the Liberals and Nationals was looking strained, both at a state and federal level. WA Nats were furious with their Liberal counterparts over a preference deal that put One Nation above the Nats in the Legislative Council. That ill-fated decision by the WA Libs reflected their unhappiness with Malcolm Turnbull's unpopularity and his unwillingness to support calls to throw more GST revenue to the West.

Of course, in the hothouse environment of the 24-hour political media, there's no time for catch-up. With another two weeks until the 11 March election, Lane picked herself up and promised herself she'd keep going, work harder. After all, she'd worked these types of hours before as ABC Sydney chief of staff. 'I'd handled it then, I'll handle it now,' she told herself.

But there was something else. 'Don't come to us in three months saying you can't handle the lack of sleep,' she'd been warned by a senior manager when she'd accepted the *AM* presenter gig. *Don't come back to us complaining you can't sleep*, cycled through her brain during those dark hours searching for sleep.

On the night of the WA election, Labor won in a landslide victory. To prepare for the Sunday-morning special election edition of *AM*, Lane went to bed at 2 a.m. She set her alarm for 3.30 a.m. For those ninety minutes, she slept, then got up and did the show without a stumble. And on Monday morning, she set the alarm again for another week of 4 a.m. starts. Interviewees couldn't make it to a 7.30 a.m. interview slot? No problem, she'd do it at 9 p.m. the day before. Work harder, always be available. *Don't complain you can't sleep.*

A week later, the sleep deficit devil came calling for payment. Federal parliament had resumed for the first time since the Coalition's defeat in the West. After presenting the Monday program, Lane stuck around parliament for a Women in Economics Network lunchtime function. The speaker was Reserve Bank Assistant Governor Dr Luci Ellis, whose nuanced take on housing affordability challenges the received wisdom that today's 'smashed avocado' generation is the first to be locked out of the property market, pointing out that the baby boomers' tendency to buy property very young has perhaps been a greater aberration, and that—surprise, surprise—divorce makes it harder to afford a home.

Lane felt tired, and ducking into the ladies', she noticed that she looked worn out. Grey, even. *Don't complain about being tired.*

Later, standing next to *The West Australian* economic editor Shane Wright, Lane suddenly felt unwell. 'My heart, oh wow, started beating furiously,' she recounts. 'I started sweating and I said to Shane, "I think I'm going to faint."' Sitting down on a chair with a glass of water did nothing to calm her racing heart. Wright, who runs marathons and is often seen checking his own heart rate while training with his dog Scully on crisp Canberra mornings, felt Lane's neck. He looked alarmed. As Wright hustled Lane downstairs to the Parliament House first-aid station, an acquaintance waved and attempted to start a conversation. 'I'm sorry,' Lane said. 'I can't talk right now. I'm having a funny turn.'

Her heart rate was 230 beats per minute. A normal resting heart rate is between sixty and 100 beats per minute. Normal aerobic exercise can safely push the heart rate to 175 beats per minute for a woman Lane's age, but anything beyond that can be considered a medical emergency. An ambulance arrived. Initially the paramedics tried to bring down her pulse naturally by asking her to blow into a device, and massaging her neck muscles to send a signal to the vagus nerve, which helps regulate blood pressure and heart rate. Her legs were elevated, but there was no change.

With her heart beating dangerously fast for more than an hour, the paramedics warned Lane that they were going to have to inject a drug to slow it and that she would feel 'a lot worse before she felt better'. She discovered the side effects of the drug, adenosine, include an 'impending sense of doom'. Strangely, this drug—along with the sting from an irukandji jellyfish, a cardiac arrest or an overdose of nutmeg—can trigger a medical symptom resembling an existential dread. For Lane, it lasted only seconds, but she had glimpsed into the abyss. She groaned out loud, no longer caring about her embarrassment at being in such a predicament in her workplace. 'Oh my God, what's happening?' she thought, later describing the sensation as a wave of doom flooding every cell in her body from her toes to her hair.

The feeling passed as her heart rate slowed, but the ordeal wasn't over. To her mortification, Lane was wheeled out of the heavy brass doors of Parliament House on a stretcher to the waiting ambulance. An alert photographer from another media organisation saw the stretcher, but not the identity of the patient, and snapped away just in case it was someone 'important'.

At Canberra Hospital, the emergency cardiologist delivered both the good news and the bad news. Lane was in good shape and her heart was undamaged by the episode that would have triggered a heart attack in someone with a less healthy muscle. But the cause of the 'supraventricular tachycardia'—a short circuit in the heart—was unknown. In the months of investigations with cardiologists that followed, it didn't occur to her that sleep deprivation could have triggered the attack. It was only later, after considering and discarding more radical options for investigation— like ablating an artery to intentionally trigger another attack—that lack of sleep appeared the most likely culprit.

A year later, Lane no longer says 'yes' to late-night prerecorded interviews; she says 'no' to a second cup of coffee or a weekday drink. She makes sure she sees the sun by exercising every day and tries not to check her phone after 8.30 p.m. For a workaholic like Lane, it's a daily challenge to know when to stop researching, stop preparing for the next day. To know when it's time to switch off.

It's been a long path to sleep recovery, including many short-lived 'fail-safe' soporifics like reading economic textbooks before bed, burning incense, wearing ear plugs and eye masks, installing block-out blinds and buying 'not-too-warm-but-not-too-cool' bedding. A daily dose of melatonin helps. But most critically, it's her realisation that no one can be 'on' all the time. 'Don't complain if you can't sleep' is no longer a career-ending threat. She's managing the hours, but now it's her heart that's calling the shots.

On a rainy Sunday afternoon over a cup of tea and later a prosecco (half a glass for Lane, a full glass for me), we talk about how these days it's up to us as individuals to impose boundaries on our work, our rest and our public lives.

Each year in every Australian state and territory, we enjoy a Labour Day public holiday without giving much thought to why it exists beyond being an excuse for a welcome long weekend at the coast, away from the usual monotony of a five-day working week. The date of the public holiday varies from state to state, so there's no nationwide ritual or tradition teaching each generation about its origins. It began with an 1856 strike by Victorian stonemasons, influenced by the beginnings of socialism in industrialised Europe, who demanded an eight-hour working day. Sure, some people still understand the significance of the arcane intertwined 8-8-8 symbol of Labour Day. Most likely they're the children of unionists, or baby boomers whose parents once took part in the annual Eight Hour March, or Labor politicians. But most of us have given up willingly and enthusiastically the observances of the eight-hour day.

Eight hours to work,
Eight hours to play,
Eight hours to sleep,
Eight bob a day.
A fair day's work,
For a fair day's pay.[11]

Now we're more likely to spend our 'eight hours' play' on Twitter, Facebook or Instagram. And insomniacs are likely to steal a slice of those 'eight hours to sleep' to

11 Nineteenth-century workers' ditty, National Museum of Australia.

stay connected during the deep, dark night. Seduced by iPhones, working from home, online purchases and GPS tracking, we've rushed to give up our personal information on how we spend our working, leisure and rest hours. We are only now beginning to realise the consequences.

The #DeleteFacebook campaign is gathering pace after the revelations of the misuse of Facebook profiles by political research firm Cambridge Analytica. How embarrassing that the tinfoil-hat conspiracy theorists were right: it's not paranoia if they really are watching you.

In hindsight, why were we so upset in 1985 by the Labor government's proposed Australia Card? So concerned about losing our personal privacy? It sought the information we currently provide through our tax file and Medicare numbers and the information we provide each year to social security agencies.

More than thirty years later, we're still resisting The Man. We resist giving information on government websites and forms like myGov and My Health Record, all the while giving it away to any online shyster who offers us the chance to 'map your run' or to win points, 'Likes' and 'chances to win!' On our phones, Fitbits and fitness tracker apps, we submit our movements from home, work, our children's school, our lover's house, our favourite dog park, local grog shop, jogging trail or nearest military installation. Our smart devices can know more about the quality of our sleep than the people who share our beds.

For insomniacs, social media is a lifeline, a connection to the rest of the world during those solitary hours of non-sleep. Switching off? Hell, no. Trust our endlessly creative and cynical youngest generation to give our anxieties a name: FOMO—fear of missing out. Slept for twelve hours straight? 'Pics or it didn't happen' is the short-hand social-media response.

Not so long ago, our everyday appliances had big, handy switches labelled 'on/off'. Suddenly and without warning, this switch evolved into an alien symbol: a single button with a circle and a short vertical line through the bottom half—presumably, the circle representing the endless 'on-ness' and the line representing 'off'. Goodness, so modern.

Now check your latest iPhone or Samsung, tablet or PC. On a PC, the off button is that minuscule button at the back. On your smart-phone there's that prominent circle, inviting you to press it with a satisfying depression of the forefinger, that will even read your finger-print. What of the vertical 'off' line? Oh, it's no longer there, replaced by discreet label-less buttons on the edge of your device. Now try turning it off. Is it really 'off' or is it just asleep? Switching off is no longer as easy as flicking a switch, is it?

Two sides of the same coin

Although both men would fiercely resist comparisons, Australia's twenty-fifth prime minister John Howard and former Australian Greens leader Bob Brown have a surprising amount in common. From the same generation (Brown is about five years Howard's junior), both of them achieving the middle-class career aspirations of their era—one a GP, the other a solicitor. Both achieving political longevity while attracting visceral reactions from opposite sides of the political spectrum. Both keeping diary notes of those difficult midnight hours as they felt the weight of history upon them.

It's 4 a.m., 12 March 2003, and Australia's Prime Minister John Howard cannot sleep. It's just over a week until the beginning of what we know now as 'the Iraq War'. Noting in his diary that the UN process towards a mandate from the Security Council had become bogged down, Howard was dismayed that the French and the Russians were stepping up their opposition to a UK- and US-led Coalition of the Willing, of which the Howard government was a staunch member. 'The momentum is all the other way,' Howard wrote early that morning.[12] It was not the first, or the last, sleepless night of his eleven-year tenure as prime minister. Nor was it the

---

12 John Howard, *Lazarus Rising: A Personal and Political Autobiography*, HarperCollins, Sydney, 2011, p. 517.

first time Howard had contemplated the existential questions of a leader.

When we speak, it's only a couple of weeks since the latest US mass shooting at Florida's Stoneman Douglas High School, which has reignited the international debate about gun control. Those frantic, grief-stricken days after the Port Arthur massacre must have been among those periods of midnight wakefulness, mustn't they? It's a free kick of a question, an invitation to wax lyrical about his most popular lasting legacy: Australia's world-leading gun-control laws. But curiously, no. It does not feature prominently in Howard's sleep story. Perhaps because he believed then, as so many of us do today, that a nationwide gun buyback was the inevitable and only course of action. Instead, Howard nominates the weight of war.

Howard's first experience of this heavy responsibility was sending Australian troops to East Timor to lead the Interfet—the UN-sanctioned International Force East Timor—in 1999, and he sent troops again to Afghanistan in 2001 after the September 11 attacks. While the liberation of East Timor and the hunt for Osama bin Laden in Afghanistan attracted broad support from the Australian public, our involvement in Iraq was a very different matter. The Iraq war remains one of the most unpopular events in our wartime history. 'I had a few relatively sleepless nights on the eve of the invasion of Iraq. And I think maybe East Timor,' he says. 'You are very conscious you have taken a decision that might end up in death for your soldiers. That weighs a lot more heavily than anything else, as it should.'

My interview with Howard is not about the rights or wrongs of Australia's military involvement during his leadership. Even after more than a decade retired from politics, Howard does not second-guess his actions while in government and has little patience with former leaders who 'self-indulgently parade a change of heart' on controversial issues.[13] However, Howard is willing to discuss those times where the burden of leadership and potential consequences of his decisions kept him awake at night. 'With the East Timor decision, events built on each other leading you inevitably to a conclusion,' he says.

---

13 Howard, p. 789.

It was not the decisions themselves that kept him awake—these 'inevitable conclusions' were reached over weeks and days after long consultation with all the key players—but rather what would happen next. 'Of course, the difficult part was what would actually happen when the troops actually entered East Timor,' he says. 'The apprehension was not about whether we'd taken the right decision or the wrong decision; the apprehension was what might happen— would they be ambushed by a rogue element of the Indonesian militia? You worry about what might happen rather than "have I taken the right decision?" because you've already been through that process.'

It's 2.40 a.m., 10 September 1996, and Greens leader Bob Brown cannot sleep. There are about 16 hours until he must deliver his maiden speech to the Senate in the new era of Howard's Australia.[14] He's wide awake and knows unless he can get some sleep, he'll be in trouble. He'll be 'tired, brain-fused, anxious'.

Unable to sleep and in despair, Brown reflected on previous generations who had lain awake at the witching hour—the soldiers in trenches, the women in the pains of child-birth. He chastises himself for lying awake worrying about being tired the next day, for being anxious about his ability to perform in a maiden speech. He reminds himself of his party's dreams: of 'forests, equality, love,

14 Bob Brown, *Optimism: Reflections on a Life of Action*, Hardie Grant Books, Melbourne, 2014, p. 85.

oceans, eternity, happiness, boundless horizons'. With all this at stake, how could he complain if he didn't sleep? 'The day will pass,' he told himself.

Over the years, putting his anxieties down on paper, and later on iPad, has helped put his sleep worries into context: the absurdity of worrying about the impact of one night without sleep on his performance in the day. On this particular night, 'It made me think about it, about people in the world with much worse situations than that, in appalling situations for whatever reason, who can't sleep,' he says. 'And in a way, how absurd, how silly it is that we find ourselves unable to sleep over some immediate discomfort … [over] anxiety to perform, but that's how it is.' Although Brown managed three hours' sleep that morning, insomnia would follow him for his next sixteen years in federal parliament. Before every big speech or demanding political event, sleep would be elusive.

Sometimes political decision-making moves fast. As with Brown's famous interjection in October 2003 on the floor of the joint sitting of parliament during the post-Iraq address by US President George W. Bush. Brown consulted fellow Greens member Kerry Nettle only the day before, and a sleepless night ensued.

Good God, most of us are preoccupied with avoiding risk, avoiding confrontation, avoiding public spectacle. Got something harsh to say? Write it down and sleep on it, because you'll feel differently in the morning. To deliberately take a course of action that invites international condemnation and death threats, and—let's be honest here—offends our polite sensibilities and the belief that we should always be nice to our guests, is not something to sleep soundly on.

It seems Howard knew Brown better than Brown might have realised. Several days before Brown had even consulted Nettle, Howard had guessed that a 'Green called Brown' could be noisy and had warned the US President, to which Bush replied, 'thanks for the warning'.[15]

As Bush addressed parliament, with Janette Howard and Laura Bush in complementary shades of blush and blue, smiling benignly from the public galleries, Brown rose to his feet. Shouting. Bush paused. A half-smile, a

---

15 Howard, p. 584.

smirk even, passed his lips. Later, after Brown
and the US President had shaken hands, even
Brown had to give credit to Bush's response:
'I love free speech!'

Since the Howard government lost the 2007
election, Australia has witnessed five changes
of prime minister—in a shorter time than
Howard's entire tenure. Could there be les-
sons about the contribution of something
as simple as sleep habits to the longevity of
a leader?

Even now, Howard is not an early-to-bed
person. He usually goes to bed between
11 p.m. and midnight and, during his prime
ministership, became famous for his 6.30 a.m.
walks in his green and gold tracksuits. He had

a routine: starting with a cup of tea at 6 a.m., a walk while listening to the radio, making his own breakfast while flicking through the papers, before a Commonwealth car arrived at the Lodge at twenty past eight in time for the 8.30 a.m. tactics meeting. Howard would not schedule any Cabinet meetings in the evening because he'd previously observed as a minister that any meeting after dinner and a couple of glasses of wine was an 'inefficient use of time'. Mostly there would be evening functions, but it was known anecdotally that Howard preferred to retire for the night after watching the ABC's *Lateline* (an impression that was 'broadly right', he admits).

Predictable? Most of the time, yes. But in Howard's view, a regular timetable was also a courtesy, as much for other people's benefit as his own. For his security detail, younger men and women who often had children. For his staff, who regularly had to be reminded to take a lunchbreak. And also for his ministers, obliged to attend endless public functions.

But how on earth do you switch off when you are the political leader of a nation, when you are responsible not just for the everyday responsibilities concerning your family and loved ones, but also for decisions that affect the lives of millions? When the buck stops with you? 'Everything becomes relative, Fleur,' Howard says. 'Once you are into the pattern, mentally you adjust to the size of the problems you face, the importance of the decisions you take.' For those of us who agonise over every career decision, every potential promotion, it's an interesting counter-argument to those midnight questions of 'what if I can't?'

These days Brown is more sanguine about those late-night and early-morning tortures we put ourselves through before we enter the public performance space. He's more relaxed about not getting the prescribed eight-hour complement, but occasionally—about once a month—he'll get up, put on a dressing gown and write when sleep eludes him.

As a GP and former parliamentarian, he's seen the costs of trying to artificially bring on that most basic of human functions. Brown was famously on duty at London's St Mary Abbot's Hospital on 18 September 1970 when Jimi Hendrix, aged twenty-seven, was brought in having died in his sleep after a cocktail of red wine and sleeping pills. But death doesn't discriminate. Brown's also seen the effects of sedatives on everyday people. As a medical student in the 1960s working at the Redfern letter-sorting centre, a worker next to him—a former truck driver—recounted driving his semitrailer up the Hume Highway at Goulburn when a ship, the *Queen Mary* with all the lights blazing, sailed across the paddocks from right to left right in front of him. As the truck driver swerved to avoid the giant passenger ship, his semitrailer crashed and he was lucky to survive. The little purple pills he'd been taking, amphetamines to stay awake and work longer, almost caused a lethal crash with a ghost ship.

Alcohol, the drug of choice in professional life, puts us to sleep, but then we wake and can't get back to sleep. 'Do you take a nip of whisky or not? Or do you put up with it? There are penalty clauses to all of these sleep-inducers,' Brown says. 'I knew this from medical school. It turns on you in the middle of the night.'

The future of parliament

It's mid-2018 and there's another debate brewing in parliament. This time over whether it's an institution fit to represent half the population: women. And some of the discussion concerns whether the family-unfriendly waking hours of parliament are part of the problem. 'It's not just about more equal representation of women and men—it's different ages, different work backgrounds and family backgrounds. It's having a parliament that looks more like the Australian people. That should be the goal that every political party sets itself and the parliament sets itself,' Labor's Deputy

Leader Tanya Plibersek told the audience on the ABC's *Q&A* program.

Contrary to popular belief, these days the Australian parliament actually has fewer sitting days and fewer late-night sittings. The hours were much worse in the 1950s and 1960s, with parliament frequently sitting until 2 or 3 a.m. Under the Whitlam government, the parliamentary sitting pattern began to assume a more manageable schedule.

Some, like Bob Brown, favour a greater overhaul of the political system, restricting sitting days to normal business hours, and compressing sitting weeks into longer blocks of time, allowing parliamentarians and their staff longer uninterrupted periods back in the electorate and at home with family. 'I think it would be better to have four or five

full days a week and have the evenings off—
all of them,' Brown says. 'If people want to,
they can have their party-room meetings and
inevitable discussions after, but earlier, and
have more sleep time at night.'

By encouraging more women and people
from diverse backgrounds to join politics,
parliament will be more representative of our
society. A more representative parliament
might help to reverse the worrying trend of
mass disengagement with mainstream politics. A more representative parliament might
inoculate Australia against the erratic swings
of undecided voters—at least that's what the
mainstream parties hope—and against decisions like the nation-shaking consequences
of Trump and Brexit. (Surely a more representative parliament would also include a

chronic procrastinator who would like to be ambitious but finds laziness, distraction and a predilection for early bedtimes get in the way of achieving #lifegoals.)

As Howard notes, Australia is no longer a country of two political tribes. Economics is no longer the dominant determinant of how people vote. Australia is no longer the 'volunteer' nation it once was—we just don't have time. Local branch meetings in the evening or at the weekend no longer attract the numbers they once did. After all, there's still work to get done, mouths to feed, lost sleep to catch up on. And politics is not a particularly attractive occupation. Think, for instance, of the unedifying twists and turns of Barnaby Joyce's private life, the 'no sex please, we're ministers' bonk ban, and Minister for Jobs and Education Michaelia Cash's slur on Opposition Leader Bill Shorten's female staffers, which may or may not be part of a grand 'Kill Bill' conspiracy. And before that, a protracted scandal over members' dual citizenship and the alleged Chinese influence over Australian politicians. Opinion polls, leadership, the date of the next federal election remain ever-present distractions. What if our elected politicians focused on getting enough sleep? Would it make a difference to the political process?

After more than three decades walking the corridors of parliament, Howard has seen it all. 'Those sorts of errors or mistakes have always occurred,' Howard says. In other words, our human traits—of ambition, of greed, of stupidity and incompetence—are as indelible as our capacity for love, patience and wisdom. And while a good night's sleep can help us make better moral decisions, it can't change human nature.

The future of sleep

A really fun thing to do at 3 a.m. is to google 'the future of sleep' for a glimpse into the dystopian future awaiting us.[16] Sheer horror will keep you awake, but at least you'll be prepared for the revolution when we are all transformed into mindless cyborgs who never sleep.

That might be a bit melodramatic. Or maybe not. Sleep devices are tipped to be the next 'big thing' in consumer electronics. We can already use Fitbits and smart watches to monitor our sleep, but the next phase of technology change will see a move from passive

---

16 Michael Q. Bullerdick, 'What "sleep" will be like in 2020, 2030 and beyond', *Van Winkles*, 4 November 2016.

monitoring to active interventions. Light-up pillows that gently wake a sleeper with the soft hues of a perfect dawn and 'smart' mattresses that self-clean and adjust to a body's temperature are just the start of this 'personal-optimisation' sleep trend. It sounds lovely.

Then the next big thing, according to futurists, is that we'll start thinking about curing the 'disease' of sleep. In the next thirty years or so, they say, we'll use sleep more deliberately to download new knowledge or skills that we don't have time to attain during our waking hours. They predict that some people will decide—or be compelled—to be genetically engineered to go without sleep. That society will be divided into the sleep 'haves' and 'have-nots'.

'Transhumanism' is the idea the human race will evolve beyond our current biological and mental limitations. It's been around since the early twentieth century, but now transhumanism is about to go mainstream. In 2017, none other than innovator Elon Musk floated the idea that humans must merge with machines if we are to remain relevant and avoid becoming little more than pets of AI entities. 'I don't love the idea of being a house cat,' Musk said.

Also in 2017, leading US futurist and transhumanism advocate Zoltan Istvan announced he would run for governor of California in November 2018. His previous tilt for the presidency in 2016 didn't go so well, but he believes California—with Silicon Valley's long obsession with 'curing' death—is ready for a transhumanist governor. After all, it voted in Arnold Schwarzenegger, the original

Terminator cyborg. 'I knew I couldn't win the election, but it was a great way to awaken many Americans to the desperate plight of our country's increasingly stifled science and innovation sector,' Istvan told *Newsweek* of his 2016 presidential campaign. 'Even libertarians like me face the real possibility that capitalism and job competition—which we always advocated for—won't survive into the next few decades because of widespread automation and the proliferation of robot workers. And what of augmenting intelligence via genetic editing— something the Chinese are leading the charge on, but most Americans seem too afraid to try? In short, what can be done to ensure the best future?' Istvan argues libertarian science advocates are needed in today's political environment, warning that technology-centric risk-takers are required as a reaction against the rise of ultra-conservative religious ideologies that threaten to stifle not just advances in AI, driverless cars, stem cell research, drones and genetic editing, but also immigration, women's rights and the environment.

Back in Australia, the idea that the natural process of sleep could soon be tweaked, controlled or eliminated by technology seems ludicrous. Howard chuckles when I ask whether democracy is up to the job of protecting our sleep. 'That really intrigues me. Imagine par-ing every hole at golf,' he says of the idea we might be able to download new skills in our sleep. 'I'm sure democracy will find a way of handling that.'

Bob Brown, who spent much of his political life lying awake at night worrying about the ecological destruction of the planet, immediately leaps on the idea of 'curing sleep'. 'We are going into terrifying technologies which define our role as human beings on a beautiful finite planet and as far as we know is the only one that has got anything like us,' he says. 'We are in an age of unbridled technology for profit, and as people are spending billions of dollars to avoid looking old, we'll have people spending billions of dollars if an answer comes along to avoid sleeping.' We are mortal beings with natural fears about existence and mortality. Sleep, he says, is part of that mortality and of being human. Sleep should be honoured, just as we should respect that we live and then we die. 'It's a little bit like winter;

it's a grounding period for the exuberance of life which follows. The next round,' he says.

To re-engineer something as elemental as sleep; well, that could only happen if democracy were bypassed or subverted. As Brown says, people just wouldn't stand for it. But the way we sleepwalked into having our personal information exploited in the Facebook/Cambridge Analytica scandal should be a cautionary tale for all of us. Will the same thing happen with transhumanism? Will we also trade away our natural sleep, that inconvenient chunk of every twenty-four hours in which we must be unconscious? Will we be so accustomed to being tired that we won't even recognise the next great moral dilemma facing our society? 'That's why I think democracy is incredibly important in defending the natural processes, including sleep,' Brown says. 'I don't know any better than anybody else why we have to sleep, but it seems to be a great institution.'

What's your sleep history?

'You know we come from a Family of Bad Sleepers,' my aunt said. Repeated in the same dark tones of an ancient prophesy, I'd heard this sort of thing before from my mother and her sisters. It's just one of our hereditary afflictions/curses, along with Dodgy Gall Bladders, Unpredictable Digestive Systems, a Tendency to Catastrophise, Bringing Bad Weather on Every Holiday and, most memorably, 'Chronic Intemperance'—as declared on the death certificate of a long-dead ancestor.

My mum, her sister and my late grandmother were all nurses. Until fairly recently, nursing was one of the few occupations available to bright Australian women of modest means. Conditioned by years of night duty, sleep—and lack of sleep—was a constant topic of family conversation. As a child, the sight of my night-shift–working mother sleepwalking on a weekday afternoon seemed hilariously eccentric. 'Have you checked Mr Arthur's IV?' she'd ask her nine-year-old daughter.

'Yes, Mum,' I'd smirk, ignoring her work-hours anxieties laid bare. During those daylight hours, she'd dream of elderly patients calling endlessly for their long-lost spouses, or of blocked stomas on the profoundly disabled children for whom my mum cared when she was not caring for her spoiled only child.

Decades later, with only occasional bouts of insomnia and as someone whose main work worry was trying not to defame someone, I'm embarrassed about my lack of empathy. 'It's not all bad,' Auntie Janice said of her chronic sleeplessness. 'You just have to not get stressed about it. I like to listen to Philip Clark.'

ABC's *Nightlife* radio program, hosted by Phil Clark and Sarah MacDonald between 10 p.m. and 2 a.m., is aimed squarely at the insomniacs of Australia and has 'everything you need to get you through the night'. From astronomy and stockmarket discussions to movie reviews and relationship advice, *Nightlife* has come to replace books and TV for my aunt, whose vision is failing. Living in a small NSW country town with her beloved cocker spaniel Pippa, those four hours in the middle of the night are a link to the rest of the world.

It's 11.30 p.m. and as Auntie Janice tunes into the 'wireless', 600 kilometres away I tune into a podcast. *Sleep with Me* is a thrice-weekly podcast of long, droning bed-time stories about perms and haircuts gone wrong, unproductive road trips, and unin-teresting *Dr Who* episodes. It's become my insomnia cure. I've become enamoured with its host, aka 'Dearest Scooter', who really does waffle on. He drifts off on tangents and into superfluous details until my brain gives up trying to follow the story and switches off. In the office the next day, my fellow insom-niacs and I trade notes on the latest Dearest Scooter podcast.

'Where did you get up to?'

'Last thing I remember is a discussion about self-addressed envelopes. You?'

'Same.'

Auntie Janice's favourite *Nightlife* segment is the quiz, and she makes a special effort to be awake to hear the listeners call in. 'The same people call in and it's like a little community. I love it,' she says.

It's an invisible community. We know who we are. Creeping through dark houses, avoiding creaking floorboards, preparing a cup of camomile tea, glass of milk, cheese and oatmeal biscuits, taking half a Sudafed, checking Twitter, sending work emails at 2 a.m., googling 'why is my eye twitching', practising yogic breathing, rehashing old regrets, making 'to do' lists, counting fucking sheep, doing a Salute to the Sun in the middle of the night. Our national dress is rumpled pyjamas, and our anthem is 'Nessun Dorma', an aria of insomniac princes and princesses who tremble with hope and with love, and watch the stars from their cold rooms.

Perhaps we all need an occasional bout of insomnia to wake us up. To take stock, to assess our weaknesses and to hear that thunderclap of midnight inspiration. Perhaps only the absence of sleep can make us appreciate its wonders.

I'm going to sleep on it.